My Diabetic All-Day Cooking Guide

An Unmissable Collection of Diabetic Drinks & Savory Recipes

Valerie Blanchard

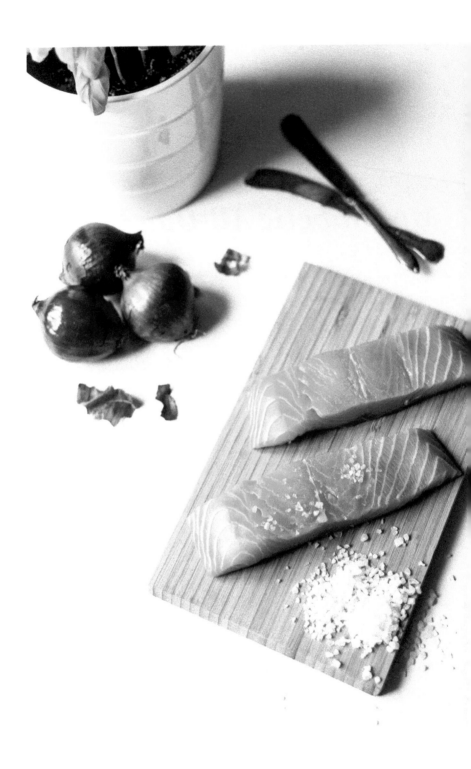

Table of Contents

6

Alkaline Green Ginger and Banana Cleansing Smoothie

Preparation Time: 15 minutes

Cooking Time: *0*

Servings: 1

Ingredients:

- One handful of kale

- one banana, frozen

- Two cups of hemp seed milk

- One inch of ginger, finely minced

- Half cup of chopped strawberries, frozen

- 1 tablespoon of agave or your preferred sweetener

Directions:

1. Mix all the **Ingredients** in a blender and mix on high speed.

2. Allow it to blend evenly.

3. Pour into a pitcher with a few decorative straws and voila you are one happy camper.

4. *Enjoy!*

Nutrition: Calories: 350; Fat: 4g; Carbohydrates: 52g; Protein: 16g

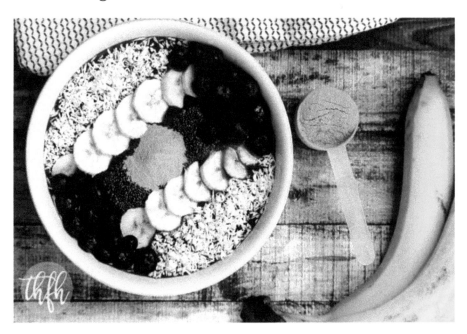

Orange Mixed Detox Smoothie

Preparation Time: 15 minutes

Cooking Time*: 0*

Servings: 1

Ingredients:

- One cup of vegies (Amaranth, Dandelion, Lettuce or Watercress)
- Half avocado
- One cup of tender-jelly coconut water
- One seville orange
- Juice of one key lime
- One tablespoon of bromide plus powder

Directions:

1. Peel and cut the Seville orange in chunks.
2. *Mix all the **Ingredients** collectively in a high-speed blender until done.*

Nutrition: Calories: 71; Fat: 1g; Carbohydrates: 12g; Protein: 2g

Cucumber Toxin Flush Smoothie

Preparation Time: 15 minutes

Cooking Time*: 0*

Servings: 1

Ingredients:

- 1 Cucumber

- 1 Key Lime

- 1 cup of watermelon (seeded), cubed

Directions*:*

1. Mix all the above **Ingredients** in a high-speed blender.

2. Considering that watermelon and cucumbers are largely water, you may not want to add any extra, however you can so if you want.

3. Juice the key lime and add into your smoothie.

4. *Enjoy!*

Nutrition: Calories: 219; Fat: 4g; Carbohydrates: 48g; Protein: 5g

Apple Blueberry Smoothie

Preparation Time: 15 minutes

Cooking Time*: 0*

Servings: 1

Ingredients:

- Half apple
- One Date
- Half cup of blueberries
- Half cup of sparkling callaloo
- One tablespoon of hemp seeds
- One tablespoon of sesame seeds
- Two cups of sparkling soft-jelly coconut water
- Half of tablespoon of bromide plus powder

Directions:

1. *Mix all of the **Ingredients** in a high-speed blender and enjoy!*

Nutrition: Calories: 167.4; Fat: 6.4g; Carbohydrates: 22.5g; Protein: 6.7g

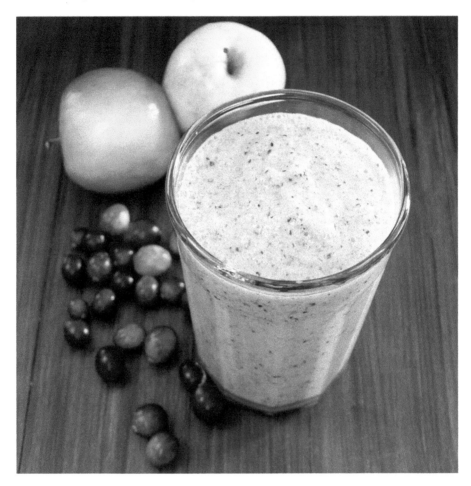

Lemon Rooibos Iced Tea

Preparation Time: 10 minutes

Cooking Time*: 0 minute*

Serving*: 4*

Ingredients:

- 4 bags natural, unflavored rooibos tea
- 4 cups boiling water
- 3 tablespoons freshly squeezed lemon juice
- 30–40 drops liquid stevia

Directions:

1. Situate tea bags into tea pot and pour the boiling water over the bags.

2. Set aside to room temperature, then refrigerate the tea until it is ice-cold.

3. Remove the tea bags. Squeeze them gently.

4. Add the lemon juice and liquid stevia to taste and stir until well mixed.

5. Serve immediately, preferably with ice cubes and some nice garnishes, like lemon wedges.

Nutrition: 70 Calories; 16g Carbohydrates; 1g Protein

Lemon Lavender Iced Tea

Preparation Time: 15minutes

Cooking Time*: 0 minute*

Serving*: 4*

Ingredients:

- 2 bags natural, unflavored rooibos tea
- 2 oz lemon chunks without peel and pith, seeds removed
- 1 teaspoon dried lavender blossoms placed in a tea ball
- 4 cups water, at room temperature
- 20–40 drops liquid stevia

Directions:

1. Place the tea bags, lemon chunks and the tightly-closed tea ball with the lavender blossoms in a 1.5 qt (1.5 l) pitcher.

2. Pour in the water.

3. Refrigerate overnight.

4. Remove the tea bags, lemon chunks and the tea ball with the lavender on the next day. Squeeze the tea bags gently to save as much liquid as possible.

5. Add liquid stevia to taste and stir until well mixed.

6. Serve immediately with ice cubes and lemon wedges.

Nutrition: 81 Calories; 12g Carbohydrates; 3g Protein

Cherry Vanilla Iced Tea

__Preparation Time:__ 12 minutes

Cooking Time*: 0 minute*

Serving*: 4*

Ingredients:

- 4 bags natural, unflavored rooibos tea

- 4 cups boiling water

- 2 tablespoons freshly squeezed lime juice

- 1–2 tablespoons cherry flavoring

- 30–40 drops (or to taste) liquid vanilla stevia

Directions:

1. Place tea bags into tea pot and pour the boiling water over the bags.

2. Put aside the tea cool down first, then refrigerate the tea until it is ice-cold.

3. Remove the tea bags. Squeeze them lightly.

4. Add the lime juice, cherry flavoring and the vanilla stevia and stir until well mixed.

5. Serve immediately, preferably with ice cubes and some nice garnishes like lime wedges and fresh cherries.

__Nutrition:__ 89 Calories; 14g Carbohydrates; 2g Protein

Elegant Blueberry Rose Water Iced Tea

Preparation Time: 12 minutes

Cooking Time*: 0 minute*

Serving*: 4*

Ingredients:

- 2 bags herbal blueberry tea
- 4 cups boiling water
- 20 drops liquid stevia
- 1 tablespoon rose water

Directions:

1. Position tea bags into tea pot and pour the boiling water over the bags.

2. Allow tea cool down first, then refrigerate the tea until it is ice-cold.

3. Remove the tea bags. Press them gently.

4. Add the liquid stevia and the rose water and stir until well mixed.

5. Serve immediately, preferably with ice cubes and some nice garnishes, like fresh blueberries or natural rose petals

Nutrition: 75 Calories; 10g Carbohydrates; 2g Protein

Melba Iced Tea

Preparation Time: 10 minutes

Cooking Time*: 0 minute*

Serving*: 4*

Ingredients:

- 1 bag herbal raspberry tea
- 1 bag herbal peach tea
- 4 cups boiling water
- 10 drops liquid peach stevia
- 20–40 drops (or to taste) liquid vanilla stevia

Directions:

1. Pour the boiling water over the tea bags.
2. Leave tea cool down on room temperature, then refrigerate the tea until it is ice-cold.
3. Remove the tea bags. Press lightly.
4. Add the peach stevia and stir until well mixed.

5. Add vanilla stevia to taste and stir until well mixed.

6. Serve immediately, preferably with ice cubes and some nice garnishes, like vanilla bean, fresh raspberries or peach slices.

Nutrition: 81 Calories; 14g Carbohydrates; 4g Protein

Merry Raspberry Cherry Iced Tea

Preparation Time: 11 minutes

Cooking Time: 0 minute

Serving: *4*

Ingredients:

- 2 bags herbal raspberry tea
- 4 cups boiling water
- 1 teaspoon stevia-sweetened cherry-flavored drink mix
- 1 teaspoon freshly squeezed lime juice
- 10–20 drops (or to taste) liquid stevia

Directions:

1. Put the tea bags into tea pot and fill in boiling water over the bags.
2. Let the tea cool down first to room temperature, then chill until it is ice-cold.

3. Discard tea bags. Squeeze them.

4. Add the cherry-flavored drink mix and the lime juice and stir until the drink mix is dissolved.

5. Add liquid stevia to taste and stir until well mixed.

6. Serve immediately, preferably with ice cubes or crushed ice and some nice garnishes, like fresh raspberries and cherries.

Nutrition: 82 Calories; 11g Carbohydrates; 4g Protein

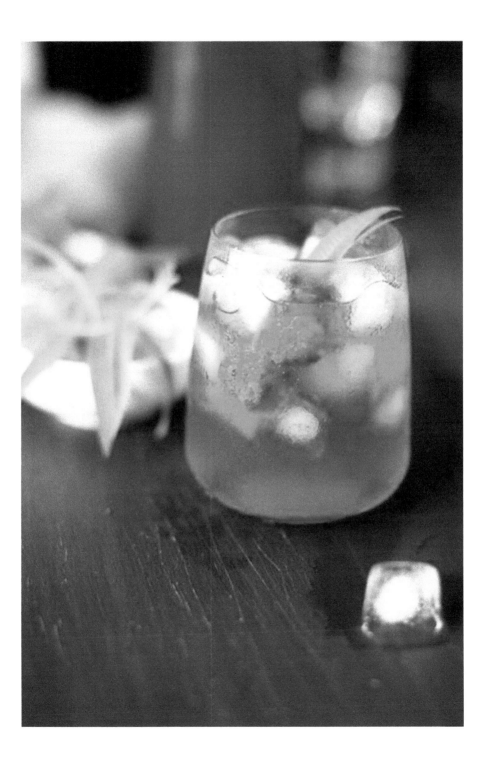

Vanilla Kissed Peach Iced Tea

Preparation Time: 13 minutes

Cooking Time*: 0 minute*

Serving*: 4*

Ingredients:

- 2 bags herbal peach tea

- 4 cups boiling water

- 1 teaspoon vanilla extract

- 1 teaspoon freshly squeezed lemon juice

- 30–40 drops (or to taste) liquid stevia

Directions:

1. Soak tea bags over boiling water.

2. Allow to cool down on room temperature, then refrigerate the tea until it is ice-cold.

3. Remove and press tea bags.

4. Add the vanilla extract and the lemon juice and stir until well mixed.

5. Add liquid stevia to taste and stir until well mixed.

6. Serve immediately, preferably with ice cubes and some nice garnishes, like peach slices.

Nutrition: 88 Calories; 14g Carbohydrates; 3g Protein

Xtreme Berried Iced Tea

Preparation Time: 10 minutes

Cooking Time*: 0 minute*

Serving*: 4*

Ingredients:

- 2 bags herbal Wild Berry Tea
- 4 cups = 950 ml boiling water
- 2 teaspoons freshly squeezed lime juice
- 40 drops berry-flavored liquid stevia
- 10 drops (or to taste) liquid stevia

Directions:

1. Submerge tea bags into boiling water.
2. Set aside to cool down, then refrigerate the tea until it is ice- cold.
3. Pull out tea bags. Squeeze.

4. Add the lime juice and the berry stevia and stir until well mixed.

5. Add liquid stevia to taste and stir until well mixed.

6. Serve immediately.

Nutrition: 76 Calories; 14g Carbohydrates; 4g Protein

Refreshingly Peppermint Iced Tea

Preparation Time: 15 minutes

Cooking Time*: 0 minute*

Serving*: 5*

Ingredients:

- 4 bags peppermint tea
- 4 cups = 950 ml boiling water
- 2 teaspoons stevia-sweetened lime-flavored drink mix
- 1 cup = 240 ml ice-cold sparkling water

Directions:

1. Immerse tea bags on boiling water.
2. Set aside before cooling until it is ice-cold.
3. Take out tea bags then press.
4. Add the lime-flavored drink mix and stir until it is properly dissolved.

5. Add the sparkling water and stir very gently.

6. Serve immediately, preferably with ice cubes, mint leaves and lime wedges.

Nutrition: 78 Calories; 17g Carbohydrates; 4g Protein

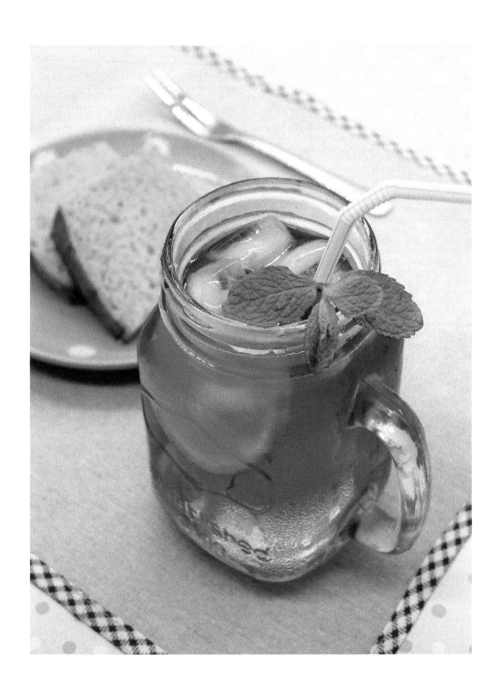

Lemongrass Mint Iced Tea

Preparation Time: 12 minutes

Cooking Time*: 0 minute*

Serving*: 4*

Ingredients:

- 1 stalk lemongrass, chopped in 1-inch
- 1/2 cup chopped, loosely packed mint sprigs
- 4 cups boiling water

Directions:

1. Put the lemongrass and the mint into tea pot and pour the boiling water over them.

2. Let cool down first to room temperature, then refrigerate until the tea is ice-cold.

3. Filter out the lemongrass and the mint.

4. Add liquid vanilla stevia to taste if you prefer some sweetness and stir until well mixed.

5. Serve immediately, preferably with ice cubes and some nice garnishes, like mint sprigs and lemongrass stalks.

Nutrition: 89 Calories; 17g Carbohydrates; 5g Protein

Spiced Tea

Preparation Time: 8 minutes

Cooking Time*: 0 minute*

Serving*: 4*

Ingredients:

- 2 bags Bengal Spice tea
- 2 teaspoons freshly squeezed lemon juice
- 1 packet zero-carb vanilla stevia
- 1 packet zero-carb stevia
- 4 cups boiling water

Directions:

1. Put the tea bags, lemon juice and the both stevia into tea pot.
2. Pour in the boiling water.
3. Put aside to cool over room temperature, then refrigerate.

4. Pull away tea bags then squeeze it.

5. Stir gently.

6. Serve immediately, preferably with ice cubes or crushed ice and some lemon wedges or slices.

Nutrition: 91 Calories; 16g Carbohydrates; 1g Protein

Infused Pumpkin Spice Latte

Preparation Time: 11 minutes

Cooking Time*: 0 minute*

Serving*: 2*

Ingredients:

- 2 cups almond milk

- ¼ cup coconut cream

- 2 teaspoons cannabis coconut oil

- ¼ cup pure pumpkin, canned

- ½ teaspoon vanilla extract

- 1 ½ teaspoon pumpkin spice

- ½ cup coconut whipped cream

- 1 pinch of salt

Directions:

1. Place all **Ingredients** except the coconut whipped cream, in pan over a medium low heat stove.

2. Whisk well and allow to simmer but don't boil!

3. Simmer for about 5 minutes.

4. Pour into mugs and serve.

__Nutrition:__ 94 Calories; 17g Carbohydrates; 3g Protein

Infused Turmeric-Ginger Tea

__Preparation Time:__ 9 minutes

Cooking Time*: 0 minute*

Serving*: 1*

Ingredients:

- 1 cup water
- ½ cup coconut milk
- 1 teaspoon cannabis oil
- ½ teaspoon ground turmeric
- ¼ cup fresh ginger root, sliced
- 1 pinch Stevia or maple syrup, to taste

Directions:

1. Combine all **Ingredients** in a small saucepan over medium heat.
2. Heat until simmer and turn heat low.
3. Take pan off the heat after 2 minutes

4. Let it cool, strain mixture into cup or mug.

Nutrition: 98 Calories; 14g Carbohydrates; 2g Protein

Infused London Fog

Preparation Time: 17 minutes

Cooking Time: *0 minute*

Serving: 2

Ingredients:

- 1 cup hot water
- 1 Earl Grey teabag
- 1 teaspoon cannabis coconut oil
- ¼ cup almond milk
- ¼ teaspoon vanilla extract
- 1 pinch Stevia or sugar, to taste

Directions:

1. Fill up half a mug with boiling water.
2. Add teabag; if you prefer your tea strong, add two.
3. Add cannabis oil and stir well.

4. Add almond milk to fill your mug and stir through with the vanilla extract

5. Use Stevia or sugar to sweeten your Earl Grey to taste.

Nutrition: 76 Calories; 14g Carbohydrates; 2g Protein

Infused Cranberry-Apple Snug

Preparation Time: 10 minutes

Cooking Time*: 0 minute*

Serving*: 1*

Ingredients:

- ½ cup fresh cranberry juice

- ½ cup fresh apple juice, cloudy

- ½ stick cinnamon

- 2 whole cloves

- ¼ lemon, sliced

- 1 pinch of Stevia or sugar, to taste

- cranberries for garnish (optional)

Directions:

1. Combine all **Ingredients** in a small saucepan over medium heat.

2. Heat until simmer and turn heat low.

3. Let it cool, strain the mixture into a mug.

4. Serve with cinnamon stick and cranberries in a mug.

__Nutrition:__ 88 Calories; 15g Carbohydrates; 3g Protein

Stomach Soother

__Preparation Time:__ 5 minutes

__Cooking Time__: 3 minutes

Servings: *1*

Ingredients:

- Agave syrup, 1 tbsp.

- Ginger tea, .5 c

- Dr. Sebi's Stomach Relief Herbal Tea

- Burro banana, 1

Directions:

1. Fix the herbal tea according to the **Directions** on the package. Set it aside to cool.

2. Once the tea is cool, place it along with all the other **Ingredients** into a blender. Switch on the blender and let it run until it is creamy.

Nutrition: Calories 25; Sugar 3g; Protein 0.3g; Fat 0.5

Sarsaparilla Syrup

Preparation Time: 15 minutes

Cooking Time*: 4 hours*

Servings: *4*

Ingredients*:*

- Date sugar, 1 c

- Sassafras root, 1 tbsp.

- Sarsaparilla root, 1 c

- Water, 2 c

Directions:

1. Firstly, add all of the **Ingredients** to a mason jar. Screw on the lid, tightly, and shake everything together. Heat a water bath up to 160. Sit the mason jar into the water bath and allow it to infuse for about two to four hours.

2. When the infusion time is almost up, set up an ice bath. Add half and half water and ice to a

bowl. Carefully take the mason jar out of the water bath and place it into the ice bath. Allow it to sit in the ice bath for 15 to 20 minutes.

3. Strain the infusion out and into another clean jar.

__Nutrition:__ Calories 37; Sugar 2g; Protein 0.4g; Fat 0.3

Dandelion "Coffee"

Preparation Time: 15 minutes

Cooking Time: 10 minutes

Servings: *4*

Ingredients:

- Nettle leaf, a pinch
- Roasted dandelion root, 1 tbsp.
- Water, 24 oz.

Directions:

1. To start, we will roast the dandelion root to help bring out its flavors. Feel free to use raw dandelion root if you want to, but roasted root brings out an earthy and complex flavor, which is perfect for cool mornings.

2. Simply add the dandelion root to a pre-warmed cast iron skillet. Allow the pieces to roast on medium heat until they start to darken in color,

and you start to smell their rich aroma. Make sure that you don't let them burn because this will ruin your teas taste.

3. As the root is roasting, have the water in a pot and allow it to come up to a full, rapid boil. Once your dandelion is roasted, add it to the boiling water with the nettle leaf. Steep this for ten minutes.

4. Strain. You can flavor your tea with some agave if you want to. Enjoy.

Nutrition: Calories 43; Sugar 1g; Protein 0.2g; Fat 0.3

Chamomile Delight

__Preparation Time:__ 5 minutes

__Cooking Time__: 10 minutes

Servings: *3*

Ingredients:

- Date sugar, 1 tbsp.

- Walnut milk, .5 c

- Dr. Sebi's Nerve/Stress Relief Herbal Tea, .25 c

- Burro banana, 1

Directions:

1. Prepare the tea according to the package **Directions** . Set to the side and allow to cool.

2. Once the tea is cooled, add it along with the above **Ingredients** to a blender and process until creamy and smooth.

Nutrition: Calories 21; Sugar 0.8g; Protein 1.0g; Fat 0.2g

Mucus Cleanse Tea

Preparation Time: 10 minutes

Cooking Time: 5 minutes

Servings: *2*

Ingredients:

- Blue Vervain

- Bladder wrack

- Irish Sea Moss

Directions:

1. Add the sea moss to your blender. This would be best as a gel. Just make sure that it is totally dry.

2. Place equal parts of the bladder wrack to the blender. Again, this would be best as a gel. Just make sure that it is totally dry. To get the best results you need to chop these by hand.

3. Add equal parts of the blue vervain to the blender. You can use the roots to increase your iron intake and **Nutrition**al healing values.

4. Process the herbs until they form a powder. This can take up to three minutes.

5. Place the powder into a non-metal pot and put it on the stove. Fill the pot half full of water. Make sure the herbs are totally immersed in water. Turn on the heat and let the liquid boil. Don't let it boil more than five minutes.

6. Carefully strain out the herbs. You can save these for later use in other recipes.

7. You can add in some agave nectar, date sugar, or key lime juice for added flavor.

*__Nutrition:__*Calories 36; Sugar 6g; Protein 0.7g; Fat 0.3g

Immune Tea

Preparation Time: 10 minutes

Cooking Time: 20 minutes

Servings: *1*

Ingredients:

- Echinacea, 1 part

- Astragalus, 1 part

- Rosehip, 1 part

- Chamomile, 1 part

- Elderflowers, 1 part

- Elderberries, 1 part

Directions:

1. Mix the herbs together and place them inside an airtight container.

2. When you are ready to make a cup of tea, place one teaspoon into a tea ball or bag, and put it in

eight ounces of boiling water. Let this sit for 20 minutes.

Nutrition: Calories 39; Sugar 1g; Protein 2g; Fat 0.6g

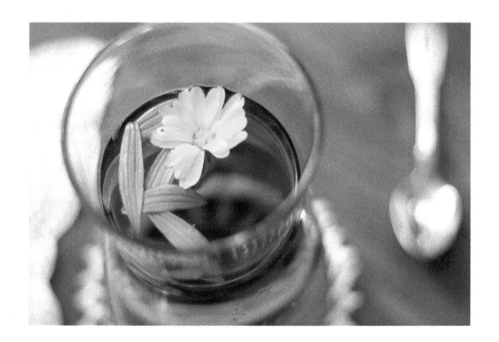

Ginger Turmeric Tea

Preparation Time: 5 minutes

Cooking Time: 15 minutes

Servings: *2*

Ingredients:

- Juice of one key lime

- Turmeric finger, couple of slices

- Ginger root, couple of slices

- Water, 3 c

Directions:

1. Pour the water into a pot and let it boil. Remove from heat and put the turmeric and ginger in. Stir well. Place lid on pot and let it sit 15 minutes.

2. While you are waiting on your tea to finish steeping, juice one key lime, and divide between two mugs.

3. Once the tea is ready, remove the turmeric and ginger and pour the tea into mugs and enjoy. If you want your tea a bit sweet, add some agave syrup or date sugar.

Nutrition: Calories 27; Sugar 5g; Protein 3g; Fat 1.0g

Tranquil Tea

Preparation Time: 5 minutes

Cooking Time: 10 minutes

Servings: *2*

Ingredients:

- Rose petals, 2 parts

- Lemongrass, 2 parts

- Chamomile, 4 parts

Directions:

1. Pour all the herbs into a glass jar and shake well to mix.

2. When you are ready to make a cup of tea, add one teaspoon of the mixture for every **Serving** to a tea strainer, ball, or bag. Cover with water that has boiled and let it sit for ten minutes.

3. If you like a little sweetness in your tea, you can add some agave syrup or date sugar.

Nutrition: Calories 35; Sugar 3.4g; Protein 2.3g; Fat 1.5g

Energizing Lemon Tea

Preparation Time: 5 minutes

Cooking Time: 15 minutes

Servings: *3*

Ingredients:

- Lemongrass, .5 tsp. dried herb

- Lemon thyme, .5 tsp. dried herb

- Lemon verbena, 1 tsp. dried herb

Directions:

1. Place the dried herbs into a tea strainer, bag, or ball and place it in one cup of water that has boiled. Let this sit 15 minutes. Carefully strain out the tea. You can add agave syrup or date sugar if needed.

Nutrition: Calories 40; Sugar 6g; Protein 2.2g; Fat 0.3

529. Respiratory Support Tea

Preparation Time: 5 minutes

Cooking Time: 18 minutes

Servings: *4*

Ingredients:

- Rosehip, 2 parts

- Lemon balm, 1 part

- Coltsfoot leaves, 1 part

- Mullein, 1 part

- Osha root, 1 part

- Marshmallow root, 1 part

Directions:

1. Place three cups of water into a pot. Place the Osha root and marshmallow root into the pot. Allow to boil. Let this simmer for ten minutes

2. Now put the remaining **Ingredients** into the pot and let this steep another eight minutes. Strain.

3. Drink four cups of this tea each day.

4. It's almost that time of year again when everyone is suffering from the dreaded cold. Then that cold turns into a nasty lingering cough. Having these **Ingredients** on hand will help you be able to get ahead of this year's cold season. When you buy your ingredient, they need to be stored in glass jars. The roots and leaves need to be put into separate jars. You can drink this tea at any time, but it is great for when you need some extra respiratory support.

__Nutrition:__ Calories 35; Sugar 3.4g; Protein 2.3g; Fat 1.5g

Thyme and Lemon Tea

Preparation Time: 5 minutes

Cooking Time: 10 minutes

Servings: *2*

Ingredients:

- Key lime juice, 2 tsp.

- Fresh thyme sprigs, 2

Directions:

1. Place the thyme into a canning jar. Boil enough water to cover the thyme sprigs. Cover the jar with a lid and leave it alone for ten minutes. Add the key lime juice. Carefully strain into a mug and add some agave nectar if desired.

Nutrition: Calories 22; Sugar 1.4g; Protein 5.3g; Fat 0.6g

Sore Throat Tea

__Preparation Time:__ 8 minutes

__Cooking Time__: 15 minutes

Servings: *4*

Ingredients:

- Sage leaves, 8 to 10 leaves

Directions:

1. Place the sage leaves into a quart canning jar and add water that has boiled until it covers the leaves. Pour the lid on the jar and let sit for 15 minutes.

2. You can use this tea as a gargle to help ease a sore or scratchy throat. Usually, the pain will ease up before you even finish your first cup. This can also be used for inflammations of the throat, tonsils, and mouth since the mucous membranes get soothed by the sage oil. A

normal dose would be between three to four cups each day. Every time you take a sip, roll it around in your mouth before swallowing it.

Nutrition: Calories 26; Sugar 2.0g; Protein 7.6g; Fat 3.2g

Autumn Tonic Tea

Preparation Time: 10 minutes

Cooking Time: 15 minutes

Servings: *2*

Ingredients:

- Dried ginger root, 1 part

- Rosehip, 1 part

- Red clover, 2 parts

- Dandelion root and leaf, 2 parts

- Mullein leaf, 2 parts

- Lemon balm, 3 parts

- Nettle leaf, 4 parts

Directions:

1. Place all of these **Ingredients** above into a bowl. Stir everything together to mix well. Put

into a glass jar with a lid and keep it in a dry place that stays cool.

2. When you want a cup of tea, place four cups of water into a pot. Let this come to a full rolling boil. Place the desired amount of tea blend into a tea strainer, ball, or bag and cover with boiling water. Let sit for 15 minutes. Strain out the herbs and drink it either cold or hot. If you like your tea sweet, add some agave syrup or date sugar.

Nutrition: Calories 43; Sugar 3.8g; Protein 6.5g; Fat 3.9g

Adrenal and Stress Health

Preparation Time: 12 minutes

Cooking Time: 20 minutes

Servings: 2

Ingredients:

- Bladder wrack, .5 c

- Tulsi holy basil, 1 c

- Shatavari root, 1 c

- Ashwagandha root, 1 c

Directions:

1. Place these **Ingredients** into a bowl. Stir well to combine.

2. Place mixture in a glass jar with a lid and store in a dry place that stays cool.

3. When you want a cup of tea, place two tablespoons of the tea mixture into a medium

pot. Pour in two cups of water. Let this come to a full rolling boil. Turn down heat. Let this simmer 20 minutes. Strain well. If you prefer your tea sweet, you can add some agave syrup or date sugar.

Nutrition: Calories 43; Sugar 2.2g; Protein 4.1g; Fat 2.3g

Lavender Tea

__Preparation Time:__ 5 minutes

__Cooking Time__: 15 minutes

Servings: *2*

Ingredients:

- Agave syrup, to taste

- Dried lavender flowers, 2 tbsp.

- Fresh lemon balm, handful

- Water, 3 c

__Directions:__

1. Pour the water in a pot and allow to boil.

2. Pour over the lavender and lemon balm. Cover and let sit for five minutes.

3. Strain well. If you prefer your tea sweet, add some agave syrup.

Nutrition: Calories 59; Sugar 6.8g; Protein 3.3g; Fat 1.6g

Scallion Sandwich

Preparation Time: 10 minutes

Cooking Time: 10 minutes

Servings: *1*

Ingredients:

- 2 slices wheat bread

- 2 teaspoons butter, low fat

- 2 scallions, sliced thinly

- 1 tablespoon of parmesan cheese, grated

- 3/4 cup of cheddar cheese, reduced fat, grated

Directions:

1. Preheat the Air fryer to 356 degrees.

2. Spread butter on a slice of bread. Place inside the cooking basket with the butter side facing down.

3. Place cheese and scallions on top. Spread the rest of the butter on the other slice of bread Put it on top of the sandwich and sprinkle with parmesan cheese.

4. Cook for 10 minutes.

Nutrition: Calorie: 154; Carbohydrate: 9g; Fat: 2.5g; Protein: 8.6g; Fiber: 2.4g

Lean Lamb and Turkey Meatballs with Yogurt

Preparation Time: 10 minutes

Servings: *4*

Cooking Time: 8 minutes

Ingredients:

- 1 egg white
- 4 ounces ground lean turkey
- 1 pound of ground lean lamb
- 1 teaspoon each of cayenne pepper, ground coriander, red chili pastes, salt, and ground cumin
- 2 garlic cloves, minced
- 1 1/2 tablespoons parsley, chopped
- 1 tablespoon mint, chopped
- 1/4 cup of olive oil

For the yogurt

- 2 tablespoons of buttermilk

- 1 garlic clove, minced

- 1/4 cup mint, chopped

- 1/2 cup of Greek yogurt, non-fat

- Salt to taste

Directions:

1. Set the Air Fryer to 390 degrees.

2. Mix all the **Ingredients** for the meatballs in a bowl. Roll and mold them into golf-size round pieces. Arrange in the cooking basket. Cook for 8 minutes.

3. While waiting, combine all the **Ingredients** for the mint yogurt in a bowl. Mix well.

4. Serve the meatballs with the mint yogurt. Top with olives and fresh mint.

Nutrition: Calorie: 154; Carbohydrate: 9g; Fat: 2.5g; Protein: 8.6g; Fiber: 2.4g

Air Fried Section and Tomato

Preparation Time: 10 minutes

Cooking Time: 5 minutes

Servings: *2*

Ingredients:

- 1 aubergine, sliced thickly into 4 disks
- 1 tomato, sliced into 2 thick disks
- 2 tsp. feta cheese, reduced fat
- 2 fresh basil leaves, minced
- 2 balls, small buffalo mozzarella, reduced fat, roughly torn
- Pinch of salt
- Pinch of black pepper

Directions:

1. Preheat Air Fryer to 330 degrees F.

2. Spray small amount of oil into the Air fryer basket. Fry aubergine slices for 5 minutes or until golden brown on both sides. Transfer to a plate.

3. Fry tomato slices in batches for 5 minutes or until seared on both sides.

4. To serve, stack salad starting with an aborigine base, buffalo mozzarella, basil leaves, tomato slice, and 1/2-teaspoon feta cheese.

5. Top of with another slice of aborigine and 1/2 tsp. feta cheese. Serve.

Nutrition: Calorie: 140.3; Carbohydrate: 26.6; Fat: 3.4g; Protein: 4.2g; Fiber: 7.3g

Cheesy Salmon Fillets

Preparation Time: 15 minutes

Cooking Time: 20 minutes

Servings: *2-3*

Ingredients: For the salmon fillets

- 2 pieces, 4 oz. each salmon fillets, choose even cuts
- 1/2 cup sour cream, reduced fat
- ¼ cup cottage cheese, reduced fat
- ¼ cup Parmigiano-Reggiano cheese, freshly grated

Garnish:

- Spanish paprika
- 1/2-piece lemon, cut into wedges

Directions:

1. Preheat Air Fryer to 330 degrees F.

2. To make the salmon fillets, mix sour cream, cottage cheese, and Parmigiano-Reggiano cheese in a bowl.

3. Layer salmon fillets in the Air fryer basket. Fry for 20 minutes or until cheese turns golden brown.

4. To assemble, place a salmon fillet and sprinkle paprika. Garnish with lemon wedges and squeeze lemon juice on top. Serve.

Nutrition: Calorie: 274; Carbohydrate: 1g; Fat: 19g; Protein: 24g; Fiber: 0.5g

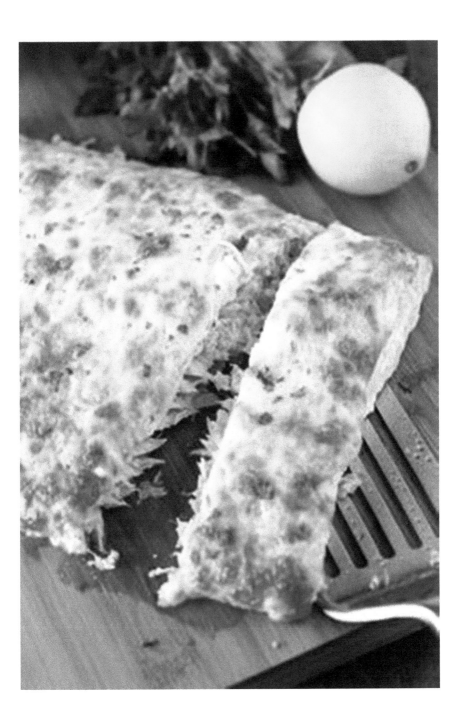

Salmon with Asparagus

Preparation Time: *5 Minutes*

Cooking Time: 10 Minutes

Servings: *3*

Ingredients:

- 1 lb. Salmon, sliced into fillets
- 1 tbsp. Olive Oil
- Salt & Pepper, as needed
- 1 bunch of Asparagus, trimmed
- 2 cloves of Garlic, minced
- Zest & Juice of 1/2 Lemon
- 1 tbsp. Butter, salted

Directions:

1. Spoon in the butter and olive oil into a large pan and heat it over medium-high heat.

2. Once it becomes hot, place the salmon and season it with salt and pepper.

3. Cook for 4 minutes per side and then cook the other side.

4. Stir in the garlic and lemon zest to it.

5. Cook for further 2 minutes or until slightly browned.

6. Off the heat and squeeze the lemon juice over it.

7. Serve it hot.

Nutrition: Calories: 409Kcal; Carbohydrates: 2.7g; Proteins: 32.8g; Fat: 28.8g; Sodium: 497mg

Shrimp in Garlic Butter

Preparation Time: *5 Minutes*

Cooking Time: 20 Minutes

Servings: *4*

Ingredients:

- 1 lb. Shrimp, peeled & deveined
- ¼ tsp. Red Pepper Flakes
- 6 tbsp. Butter, divided
- 1/2 cup Chicken Stock
- Salt & Pepper, as needed
- 2 tbsp. Parsley, minced
- 5 cloves of Garlic, minced
- 2 tbsp. Lemon Juice

Directions:

1. Heat a large bottomed skillet over medium-high heat.

2. Spoon in two tablespoons of the butter and melt it. Add the shrimp.

3. Season it with salt and pepper. Sear for 4 minutes or until shrimp gets cooked.

4. Transfer the shrimp to a plate and stir in the garlic.

5. Sauté for 30 seconds or until aromatic.

6. Pour the chicken stock and whisk it well. Allow it to simmer for 5 to 10 minutes or until it has reduced to half.

7. Spoon the remaining butter, red pepper, and lemon juice to the sauce. Mix.

8. Continue cooking for another 2 minutes.

9. Take off the pan from the heat and add the cooked shrimp to it.

10. Garnish with parsley and transfer to the **Serving** bowl.

11. Enjoy.

Nutrition: Calories: 307Kcal; Carbohydrates: 3g; Proteins: 27g; Fat: 20g; Sodium: 522mg

Cobb Salad

Keto & Under 30 Minutes

Preparation Time: *5 Minutes*

__Cooking Time__: 5 Minutes

Servings: *1*

Ingredients:

- 4 Cherry Tomatoes, chopped

- ¼ cup Bacon, cooked & crumbled

- 1/2 of 1 Avocado, chopped

- 2 oz. Chicken Breast, shredded

- 1 Egg, hardboiled

- 2 cups Mixed Green salad

- 1 oz. Feta Cheese, crumbled

Directions:

1. Toss all the **Ingredients** for the Cobb salad in a large mixing bowl and toss well.

2. Serve and enjoy it.

Nutrition: Calories: 307KcalC; arbohydrates: 3g; Proteins: 27g; Fat: 20g; Sodium: 522mg

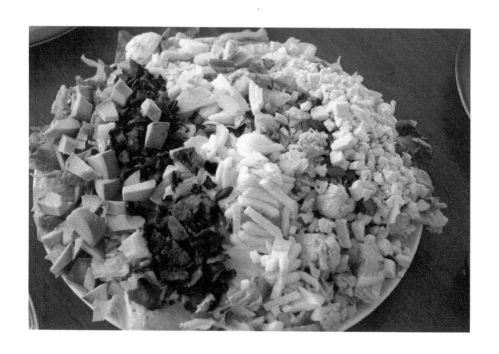

Seared Tuna Steak

Preparation Time: *10 Minutes*

Cooking Time: 10 Minutes

Serving Size*: 2*

Ingredients:

- 1 tsp. Sesame Seeds
- 1 tbsp. Sesame Oil
- 2 tbsp. Soya Sauce
- Salt & Pepper, to taste
- 2 × 6 oz. Ahi Tuna Steaks

Directions:

1. Seasoning the tuna steaks with salt and pepper. Keep it aside on a shallow bowl.

2. In another bowl, mix soya sauce and sesame oil.

3. pour the sauce over the salmon and coat them generously with the sauce.

4. Keep it aside for 10 to 15 minutes and then heat a large skillet over medium heat.

5. Once hot, keep the tuna steaks and cook them for 3 minutes or until seared underneath.

6. Flip the fillets and cook them for a further 3 minutes.

7. Transfer the seared tuna steaks to the **Serving** plate and slice them into 1/2-inch slices. Top with sesame seeds.

Nutrition: Calories: 255Kcal; Fat: 9g; Carbohydrates: 1g; Proteins: 40.5g; Sodium: 293mg

Beef Chili

Preparation Time: *10 Minutes*

Cooking Time: 20 Minutes

Serving Size*: 4*

Ingredients:

- 1/2 tsp. Garlic Powder
- 1 tsp. Coriander, grounded
- 1 lb. Beef, grounded
- 1/2 tsp. Sea Salt
- 1/2 tsp. Cayenne Pepper
- 1 tsp. Cumin, grounded
- 1/2 tsp. Pepper, grounded
- 1/2 cup Salsa, low-carb & no-sugar

Directions:

1. Heat a large-sized pan over medium-high heat and cook the beef in it until browned.

2. Stir in all the spices and cook them for 7 minutes or until everything is combined.

3. When the beef gets cooked, spoon in the salsa.

4. Bring the mixture to a simmer and cook for another 8 minutes or until everything comes together.

5. Take it from heat and transfer to a **Serving** bowl.

Nutrition: Calories: 229Kcal; Fat: 10g; Carbohydrates: 2g; Proteins: 33g; Sodium: 675mg

Greek Broccoli Salad

Preparation Time: 10 Minutes

Cooking Time: 15 Minutes

Servings: *4*

Ingredients:

- 1 ¼ lb. Broccoli, sliced into small bites
- ¼ cup Almonds, sliced
- 1/3 cup Sun-dried Tomatoes
- ¼ cup Feta Cheese, crumbled
- ¼ cup Red Onion, sliced

For the dressing:

- 1/4 cup Olive Oil
- Dash of Red Pepper Flakes
- 1 Garlic clove, minced
- ¼ tsp. Salt
- 2 tbsp. Lemon Juice
- 1/2 tsp. Dijon Mustard

- 1 tsp. Low Carb Sweetener Syrup

- 1/2 tsp. Oregano, dried

Directions:

1. Mix broccoli, onion, almonds and sun-dried tomatoes in a large mixing bowl.

2. In another small-sized bowl, combine all the dressing **Ingredients** until emulsified.

3. Spoon the dressing over the broccoli salad.

4. Allow the salad to rest for half an hour before serving.

Nutrition: Calories: 272Kcal; Carbohydrates: 11.9g; Proteins: 8g; Fat: 21.6g; Sodium: 321mg

Cheesy Cauliflower Gratin

Preparation Time: *5 Minutes*

Cooking Time: 25 Minutes

Servings: 6

Ingredients:

- 6 deli slices Pepper Jack Cheese
- 4 cups Cauliflower florets
- Salt and Pepper, as needed
- 4 tbsp. Butter
- 1/3 cup Heavy Whipping Cream

Directions:

1. Mix the cauliflower, cream, butter, salt, and pepper in a safe microwave bowl and combine well.

2. Microwave the cauliflower mixture for 25 minutes on high until it becomes soft and tender.

3. Remove the **Ingredients** from the bowl and mash with the help of a fork.

4. Taste for seasonings and spoon in salt and pepper as required.

5. Arrange the slices of pepper jack cheese on top of the cauliflower mixture and microwave for 3 minutes until the cheese starts melting.

6. Serve warm.

Nutrition: Calories: 421Kcal; Carbohydrates: 3g; Proteins: 19g; Fat: 37g; Sodium: 111mg

Strawberry Spinach Salad

Preparation Time: *5 Minutes*

Cooking Time: 10 Minutes

Servings: *4*

Ingredients:

- 4 oz. Feta Cheese, crumbled
- 8 Strawberries, sliced
- 2 oz. Almonds
- 6 Slices Bacon, thick-cut, crispy and crumbled
- 10 oz. Spinach leaves, fresh
- 2 Roma Tomatoes, diced
- 2 oz. Red Onion, sliced thinly

Directions:

1. For making this healthy salad, mix all the **Ingredients** needed to make the salad in a large-sized bowl and toss them well.

Nutrition: Calories: 255kcal; Fat: 16g; Carbohydrates: 8g; Proteins: 14g; Sodium: 27mg

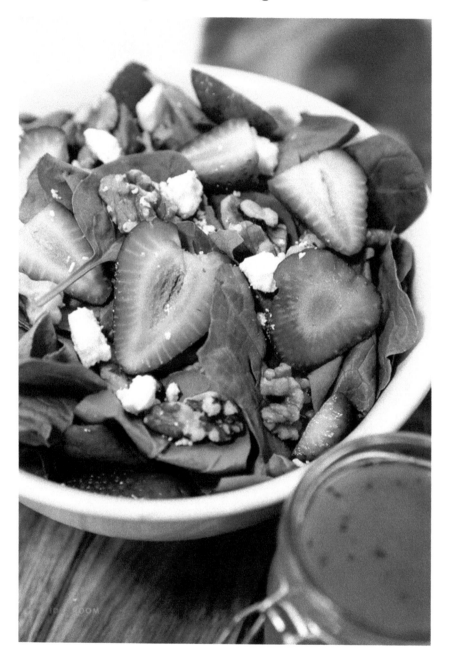

Misto Quente

__Preparation Time:__ 5 minutes

__Cooking Time__: 10 minutes

Servings: *4*

Ingredients:

- 4 slices of bread without shell
- 4 slices of turkey breast
- 4 slices of cheese
- 2 tbsp. cream cheese
- 2 spoons of butter

Directions:

1. Preheat the air fryer. Set the timer of 5 minutes and the temperature to 200C.

2. Pass the butter on one side of the slice of bread, and on the other side of the slice, the cream cheese.

3. Mount the sandwiches placing two slices of turkey breast and two slices cheese between the breads, with the cream cheese inside and the side with butter.

4. Place the sandwiches in the basket of the air fryer. Set the timer of the air fryer for 5 minutes and press the power button.

__Nutrition:__ Calories: 340; Fat: 15g; Carbohydrates: 32g; Protein: 15g; Sugar: 0g; Cholesterol: 0mg

Garlic Bread

Preparation Time: 10 minutes

Cooking Time: 15 minutes

Servings: *4-5*

Ingredients:

- 2 stale French rolls
- 4 tbsp. crushed or crumpled garlic
- 1 cup of mayonnaise
- Powdered grated Parmesan
- 1 tbsp. olive oil

Directions:

1. Preheat the air fryer. Set the time of 5 minutes and the temperature to 2000C.
2. Mix mayonnaise with garlic and set aside.
3. Cut the baguettes into slices, but without separating them completely.

4. Fill the cavities of equals. Brush with olive oil and sprinkle with grated cheese.

5. Place in the basket of the air fryer. Set the timer to 10 minutes, adjust the temperature to 1800C and press the power button.

Nutrition: Calories: 340; Fat: 15g; Carbohydrates: 32g; Protein: 15g Sugar: 0g; Cholesterol: 0mg

Bruschetta

Preparation Time: 5 minutes

Cooking Time: 10 minutes

Servings: *2*

Ingredients:

- 4 slices of Italian bread
- 1 cup chopped tomato tea
- 1 cup grated mozzarella tea
- Olive oil
- Oregano, salt, and pepper
- 4 fresh basil leaves

Directions:

1. Preheat the air fryer. Set the timer of 5 minutes and the temperature to 2000C.

2. Sprinkle the slices of Italian bread with olive oil. Divide the chopped tomatoes and

mozzarella between the slices. Season with salt, pepper, and oregano.

3. Put oil in the filling. Place a basil leaf on top of each slice.

4. Put the bruschetta in the basket of the air fryer being careful not to spill the filling. Set the timer of 5 minutes, set the temperature to 180C, and press the power button.

5. Transfer the bruschetta to a plate and serve.

Nutrition: Calories: 434; Fat: 14g; Carbohydrates: 63g; Protein: 11g; Sugar: 8g; Cholesterol: 0mg

Cream Buns with Strawberries

__Preparation Time:__ 10 minutes

__Cooking Time__: 12 minutes

Servings: 6

Ingredients:

- 240g all-purpose flour

- 50g granulated sugar

- 8g baking powder

- 1g of salt

- 85g chopped cold butter

- 84g chopped fresh strawberries

- 120 ml whipping cream

- 2 large eggs

- 10 ml vanilla extract

- 5 ml of water

Directions:

1. Sift flour, sugar, baking powder and salt in a large bowl. Put the butter with the flour with the use of a blender or your hands until the mixture resembles thick crumbs.

2. Mix the strawberries in the flour mixture. Set aside for the mixture to stand. Beat the whipping cream, 1 egg and the vanilla extract in a separate bowl.

3. Put the cream mixture in the flour mixture until they are homogeneous, and then spread the mixture to a thickness of 38 mm.

4. Use a round cookie cutter to cut the buns. Spread the buns with a combination of egg and water. Set aside

5. Preheat the air fryer, set it to 180C.

6. Place baking paper in the preheated inner basket.

7. Place the buns on top of the baking paper and cook for 12 minutes at 180C, until golden brown.

Nutrition: Calories: 150; Fat: 14g; Carbohydrates: 3g; Protein: 11g; Sugar: 8g; Cholesterol: 0mg